HOW TO EAT MINDFULLY

EATING TACTICS FOR WORKING FROM
HOME

AHMED .R

Contents

CHAPTER ONE

INTRODUCTION

The idea of mindfulness has drawn a lot of attention in the fast-paced world of today, particularly in the fields of wellness and nutrition. Eating mindfully has become more important than ever due to the shift toward remote work and the rise in time spent at home. You may improve your general well-being and relationship with food by introducing mindfulness into your eating habits, whether you're working, studying, or just lounging around the house.

Comprehending Mindful Eating

The practice of mindful eating involves focusing entirely on the internal and exterior aspects of the eating and drinking experience. It entails developing a closer relationship with the food you eat, being fully present in the moment, and recognizing your thoughts, feelings, and sensations without passing judgment.

Advantages of Intentional Eating

Practicing mindful eating has several advantages for your emotional, mental, and physical well-being:

Better Digestion: You may help your body digest food more effectively and lessen digestive discomfort like bloating and indigestion by taking your time and enjoying every bite.

Enhanced Satisfaction: You'll feel more satisfied and enjoy meals more when you practice mindful eating, which enables you to identify and react to your body's signals of hunger and fullness.

Weight management: By practicing mindful eating, you can better understand your body's requirements and maintain a healthy weight without resorting to severe diets.

Decreased Stress: By encouraging a tranquil and thoughtful approach to mealtimes, mindful eating lowers stress levels and encourages relaxation.

Increased Food Appreciation: You can gain a greater appreciation for the sustenance that food offers by using all of your senses to thoroughly experience the taste, texture, and scent of food.

Advice for Mindful Eating at Home

Establish a Calm Environment: Assign an area for meals that isn't cluttered with work-related objects or electronics. Play some relaxing music or turn down the lights to create a relaxing mood.

Practice Gratitude: Give thanks for the food on your plate and the labor of love that went into its preparation for a moment before you eat. This small gesture can improve your eating experience and help you develop a good outlook.

Eat Without Distractions: Steer clear of multitasking when eating, such as browsing through your phone or watching TV. Rather, concentrate just on the process of eating, savoring every bite's flavors, textures, and sensations.

Chew Carefully: Give each bite your full attention to ensure that the flavors fully develop and to facilitate the digestive process. Before swallowing, try to chew each bite for at least 20 to 30 seconds.

Pay Attention to Your Body: Pay attention to the signals your body sends out regarding hunger and fullness. Eat when you're hungry and stop when you're full. Take a moment to pause between bites and pay attention to your body's messages to avoid overindulging.

Engage in Mindful Snacking: If you discover that you frequently reach for snacks during the day, handle these situations mindfully. Consider if you're eating because you're bored or stressed out or if you're actually hungry.

Involve Your Senses: Focus on the flavors, textures, scents, and colors of your meal as well as other sensory components of eating. Observe how you feel after each bite and how various foods affect your body.

Your body, mind, and soul can be nourished and your relationship with food can be transformed by including mindful eating techniques into your daily routine. Even when juggling the responsibilities of a home-based lifestyle, you may embrace a better, more balanced approach to nutrition and relish the small pleasures of eating by practicing mindfulness and presence throughout mealtimes.

The meaning of awareness

Concentrated attention on the here and now, free from judgment or attachment to ideas, feelings, or sensations as they arise, is the hallmark of mindfulness. It entails purposefully paying open, curious, and accepting attention to one's ideas, feelings, physical sensations, and environment. Deep breathing, body scans, and meditation are some of the methods used in mindfulness practices to develop increased awareness and present in day-to-day living. In addition to promoting a better awareness of oneself, mindfulness aims to lower stress and anxiety, strengthen emotional control, and promote general wellbeing.

Comprehending Mindful Eating

In order to experience food in a more profound and meaningful way, mindful eating entails using all of the senses when eating, as well as being totally present and attentive throughout. It's about your connection with food and how you eat in addition to what you eat. Key concepts in mindful eating are as follows:

Present Moment Awareness: Mindful eating places a strong emphasis on being totally present in the moment when consuming food and focusing on all of its sensory aspects, including taste, texture, scent, and appearance.

Observing your thoughts, feelings, and physical experiences associated with eating without passing judgment or offering criticism is known as non-judgmental observation. This entails embracing whatever comes up while eating without categorizing it as good or negative.

Attunement to Hunger and Fullness: Rather than relying on outside cues or emotional triggers, mindful eating promotes tuning into your body's signals of hunger and fullness, eating when you're physically hungry, and stopping when you're satisfied.

Savoring Every mouthful: Eating mindfully is giving each mouthful of food careful attention and taking the time to chew it slowly and thoroughly so that you can fully absorb its flavors and sensations.

Being aware of the factors that may cause emotional eating, distinguishing between emotional and physical hunger, and coming up with non-food alternatives to deal with emotions are all part of being aware of emotional eating.

Gratitude and Appreciation: Mindful eating frequently includes expressions of gratitude for the food's origins as well as appreciation for the sustenance it offers your body.

Cultivation of Mindful Habits: Mindful eating encourages thoughtful grocery shopping, meal planning, and preparation. It goes beyond the concept of individual meals to include general eating habits and food choices.

In general, mindful eating encourages a more positive, balanced relationship with food and increases feelings of pleasure, contentment, and wellbeing during the eating process. By encouraging more deliberate and attentive eating, it can also assist general health objectives including mental well-being, digestion, and weight management.

Difficulties of Mindful Eating at Home

Although mindful eating at home has many advantages, there are several difficulties that people could run into. The following are some typical obstacles to mindful eating at home:

Distractions: TV, electronics, family, and housework are just a few examples of the many distractions that can be found in a home, which can make it difficult to be aware when eating.

Work-Life Balance: People may find it difficult to set aside specific times for meals without letting stress or other distractions from work get in the way of their eating. This is because the lines between work and home life are becoming increasingly blurred.

Emotional Eating Triggers: Spending time at home might set off emotional eating reactions or patterns, such as stress eating, nibbling out of boredom, or turning to food as a coping tool, all of which can interfere with mindful eating.

Convenience foods and snacking: People may be tempted to eat mindlessly or impulsively, disregarding hunger cues or nutritional value, due to the availability of processed and convenient foods at home and easy access to snacks throughout the day.

Mealtime Structure: It might be difficult to retain awareness and intentionality throughout meals if there are inconsistent mealtime routines or unpredictable timetables at home. This can interfere with the development of mindful eating habits.

Social Influences: Eating with relatives or housemates who might not follow a mindful eating regimen or who have different food preferences might affect how each person eats and take away from the thoughtful nature of mealtimes.

Limited Food Options: People may have limited options when it comes to what they can eat at home. This can have an effect on the variety and caliber of meals as well as the pleasure of mindful eating, depending on things like financial limitations or ingredient availability.

External Stressors: It can be difficult to concentrate on the present moment and practice mindful eating when faced with external stressors like money worries, relationship problems, or health concerns. These can also cause a heightened level of anxiety or distraction during meals.

CHAPTER TWO

Cultural and societal Norms: Beliefs about food and eating practices in the household may be at odds with mindful eating principles, causing people to put societal pressure ahead of their own personal mindfulness objectives.

Absence of Accountability: People may find it difficult to sustain regular mindful eating practices at home if there is no external accountability or support structure in place, particularly if they are not receiving encouragement or support from others.

It takes awareness, intentionality, and practice to deal with these issues. Setting limits for mealtimes, establishing a mindful eating space, engaging in self-compassion exercises, and asking for help from others are some of the strategies that can assist people in overcoming challenges and developing a more mindful home dining environment.

Advice for Mindful Eating at Home

You may improve your general well-being and change your connection with food by adopting mindful eating practices at home. The following advice will assist you in developing awareness at mealtimes in your home:

Establish a Mindful Eating Environment: Make your dining space feel calm and welcoming to start the process of mindful eating. To encourage calm and concentration, turn down the lights, turn on some relaxing music, or light a candle.

Reduce Distractions: During mealtimes, keep distractions to a minimum, such as electronic devices, television, and work-related materials. Just concentrate on the act of eating, and use all of your senses in this instant.

Use All Your Senses: Examine the look, feel, and aroma of your food for a moment before taking a mouthful. As you get ready to eat, take note of the scents, colors, and forms, as well as any new experiences that come to mind.

Practice Gratitude: Give thanks for the food you're eating by taking a minute to recognize the labor-intensive processes involved in its cultivation, preparation, and serving. Develop gratitude for the sustenance it offers your body and mind.

Chew Carefully: Take your time eating, giving each bite careful chewing before swallowing. Savor the flavors as they emerge by paying attention to the taste, texture, and experience of every bite.

Pay Attention to Your Body's Cues About Hunger and Fullness: Use these cues to help you make mindful eating choices. Eat only when you are physically hungry and stop when you are full, without depending on mood swings or other outside cues.

Eat Conscientiously, Not Mindlessly: Take note of your eating patterns and steer clear of mindless eating practices like eating straight from the box, nibbling while preoccupied, or snacking out of boredom.

Practice Portion Control: Pay attention to your body's satiety signals to prevent overindulging and serve yourself reasonable portion amounts. Throughout the meal, pay attention to how your body feels, and stop eating when you're satisfied but not overstuffed.

Take a moment to check in with yourself and gauge your degree of hunger in between bites. Before you continue eating, set down your utensils, inhale deeply, and pay attention to any feelings or sensations that surface.

After you've completed your dinner, pause to think back on your dining experience. Take note of your body's sensations, any ideas or feelings that surfaced, and any realizations you had while engaging in mindful eating.

You can develop a greater feeling of awareness, appreciation, and contentment with your eating habits at home by implementing these suggestions into your daily routine. Eating mindfully builds a stronger bond between you and the food you eat, as well as nourishing your body and soul

.

Methods for Developing Intentionality During Meals

Developing mindfulness when eating entails paying close attention to and being aware of the whole eating process. The following strategies can assist you in cultivating mindfulness when eating:

Initiate your meal with mindful breathing by taking a few deep breaths to ground yourself and focus on the here and now. Using your breath as an anchor to develop awareness, pay attention to the sensations of your breath coming into and going out of your body.

Body Scan: Before you take the first mouthful, look over your entire body, head to toe. As you are ready to eat, pay attention to any spots that feel tight or uncomfortable and give yourself permission to let go of those feelings.

Eat more slowly, chewing each bite carefully, and take time to appreciate the flavors and textures of your food. Set down your cutlery in between mouthful and take moments to savor the flavors and textures of your food.

Involve Your Senses: Focus on the flavors, textures, scents, and colors of your meal as well as other sensory components of eating. Savor every bite of your food and take note of how it tastes, looks, and feels in your mouth.

Practice non-judgmental awareness by paying attention to your eating-related thoughts, feelings, and sensations without passing judgment or offering criticism. When judgments come to mind, acknowledge them and allow them to pass without becoming entangled in them.

Mindful Eating Meditation: Prior to eating, take a few minutes to practice mindfulness meditation. Shut your eyes and concentrate on your breathing. Then, while you carefully chew each bite, turn your attention to the feelings of your food.

Gratitude Practice: Make an effort to be grateful for the food you eat by taking a moment to recognize its sources and the labor-intensive processes involved in its growth, preparation, and serving. Give thanks for all the nutrition it gives your body and mind.

Check In With Hunger and Fullness: Pay attention to your body's signals of hunger and fullness during the course of your meal. Observe any shifts in your appetite and eat only when you are physically hungry, not because of other influences or feelings.

Journaling Your Mindful Eating Experiences: Maintain a journal to record your mindful eating experiences. Jot down your observations, realizations, and difficulties as well as your thoughts about the benefits of practicing mindfulness at meals for your general wellbeing.

Exercise Mindful Gratitude: As you close your dinner, give thanks for the food you've consumed and the sustenance it has provided. Consider how all living things have a connection to each other during the food production process.

You can develop mindfulness and strengthen your bond with the food you eat by implementing these tactics into your eating habit. This will increase your awareness, appreciation, and enjoyment of the eating experience.

Overcoming Typical Obstacles

Being aware of these typical obstacles and having the patience and willingness to form new habits are necessary for practicing mindful eating. Here are some methods to deal with some typical roadblocks:

Distractions: Set apart mealtimes as a holy time where no electronics, TVs, or work-related duties are allowed. Establish a relaxing atmosphere so that you can enjoy your meal to the fullest.

Emotional Eating: Identify the emotional triggers that cause eating and create healthy coping strategies to address underlying feelings without using food, such journaling, deep breathing, or taking walks.

Convenience Foods: Arrange and cook your meals ahead of time so that healthier options are always on hand. Keep healthful foods in your kitchen that encourage mindful eating and reduce the amount of highly processed or alluring snacks there are.

Unregular Meal Times: Even in a flexible home setting, try to maintain regular meal times. In order to prioritize eating at regular intervals and prevent protracted periods of hunger, set reminders if necessary.

Social Influences: Ask family members or roommates to support you in establishing a mindful eating environment by sharing your mindful eating objectives with them. Set a good example and promote distraction-free shared meals.

Absence of Accountability: Find an accountability partner or enroll in a mindful eating group to exchange experiences and offer support to one another. You can make your commitment to mindful eating stronger by interacting with like-minded people.

Cultural Norms: Honor cultural customs while modifying mindful eating techniques to suit individual objectives and ideals. Strike a balance between adhering to cultural customs and implementing mindful eating ideas into everyday life.

External Stressors: Learn stress-reduction strategies to deal with outside pressures that can prevent you from eating mindfully, such yoga, meditation, or mindfulness activities. Make self-care a priority to improve emotional stability and resilience.

Negative Self-Talk: When faced with obstacles in mindful eating, cultivate self-compassion and engage in non-judgmental awareness. Acknowledge that failures are a necessary component of learning and seize the chance to improve and reflect on yourself.

Consistency and Persistence: Accept the fact that mindful eating is a continuous activity that calls for perseverance and patience. Even in the face of setbacks, recognize your progress and celebrate little triumphs as you continue to hone your mindful eating techniques.

You may overcome typical hurdles and develop a more thoughtful and fulfilling relationship with food at home by putting these ideas into practice and tackling problems with inquiry and resilience.

Including Mindful Eating in Everyday Living

Including intentionality and mindful awareness in your eating routines and habits is the first step towards integrating mindful eating into your daily life. Here's how to include mindful eating into your daily routine:

Start Your Day Mindfully: Whether it's a quick meditation, a deep breathing exercise, or just making the decision to eat mindfully all day, start your day with a moment of awareness.

Plan Ahead: Give yourself enough time to carefully examine nutrient-dense foods that will support your overall health and nourishment when you plan your meals and snacks. Cook mindfully and carefully, paying attention to the tastes, textures, and hues of the ingredients.

Shop for groceries with mindfulness: Approach the experience with awareness when you go food shopping. When choosing whole, fresh foods, take your time and pay attention to how each item feels in your hands—from the texture of the package to the weight of the produce.

CHAPTER THREE

Make Rituals Around Meals: To remind yourself when it's time to eat mindfully, create rituals or routines around mealtimes. This may include saying a prayer of appreciation before you eat, carefully setting the table, or lighting a candle.

Eat Without Distractions: Put electronics away, switch off screens, and concentrate just on the act of eating to reduce distractions during meals. Enjoy the experience to the fullest, taking in the flavors and textures of your meal with each bite.

Adopt a Mindful Snacking Approach: Rather than mindlessly chewing while preoccupied, approach snacking with mindfulness by selecting healthful snacks and eating them thoughtfully.

Before grabbing a food, stop for a moment and assess how hungry you are.

Pay Attention to Your Body: Throughout the day, pay attention to your body's signals of hunger and fullness. Eat when you're hungry and stop when you're full. Instead of following strict meal plans, follow your body's natural cycles when eating.

Practice thankfulness: Before, during, and after meals, express your thankfulness for the food you eat and the nourishment it brings. Consider where your food comes from and the work that went into cultivating, cooking, and presenting it.

Taking a few deep breaths before eating, chewing carefully, and enjoying every bite are all ways to practice mindful eating while on the go or in a rush. Discover moments of presence and quiet among the everyday grind.

Think and Grow: At the end of each day, consider the mindful eating experiences you've had. Take note of any revelations, difficulties, or opportunities for improvement, and utilize this reflection to guide your future work.

You may develop a more thoughtful attitude to feeding your body and soul, strengthen your relationship with food, and improve your general well-being by incorporating these mindful eating techniques into your everyday life.

It takes commitment, self-awareness, and a dedication to gradually cultivate mindful habits to maintain consistency and development in mindful eating. Here are some tips to help you maintain consistency and advance steadily in your mindful eating journey:

Establish Clear aims: Make sure your aims and goals for mindful eating are clear. Describe the practice's purpose and the reasons it's significant to you. Staying motivated and focused is made easier when you have a clear purpose.

Establish a Routine: Make mealtimes and mindful eating habits part of a regular schedule. Establish regular mealtimes and develop routines or habits that alert you when it's time to eat with awareness.

Develop Mindful Awareness: Don't limit your practice to mealtimes; make it a habit in all facets of your life. To improve your capacity for present-moment awareness, include mindfulness exercises into your everyday routine, such as body scans, meditation, or deep breathing.

Start Small: One meal or snack a day should include mindful eating at first. Add more meals and snacks to the routine progressively as you get more accustomed to it. It's easier to stay consistent and avoid overwhelm by starting small.

Prioritize Progress Over Perfection: Recognize that developing the skill of mindful eating takes time, and that progress may be made gradually. Embrace each step of your journey and concentrate on creating incremental, sustainable changes rather than striving for perfection.

Exercise Self-Compassion: When you have difficulties or failures in your mindful eating practice, treat yourself with kindness and gentleness. Give yourself compassion and understanding instead of self-criticism, acknowledging that growth and learning require time.

Remain Engaged: Exert yourself to be totally focused on your meal, especially in the face of interruptions or hectic plans. Every time your thoughts stray, bring them back to the present and concentrate on the feelings associated with eating.

Regularly Reflect: Give your experiences with mindful eating some thought. Examine your eating habits for any patterns or trends, and note any areas that could want improvement. Make the most of this reflection to advance your knowledge and development.

Seek Support: Be in the company of encouraging people who can hold you accountable or who share your ambitions. Become a part of a mindful eating community, consult a mindfulness coach, or enlist the help of loved ones who respect and comprehend your path.

Remain Adaptive and Flexible: Show that you are prepared to modify your mindful eating routine to fit your evolving requirements and situation. Because life is unpredictable, there may be moments when it seems difficult to be consistent. Even when you're busy or under pressure, maintain your flexibility and come up with inventive methods to include mindful eating into your everyday routine.

You may stay consistent and move closer to creating a more thoughtful and healthful relationship with food by implementing these techniques into your mindful eating routine. Recall that every deliberate decision you make moves you closer to your objectives and that consistency is essential.

Summary

In summary, mindful eating promotes a closer relationship with food, improves general wellbeing, and provides a transforming method of feeding the body and the mind. We can develop awareness, gratitude, and intentionality in the way we take care of ourselves by incorporating mindfulness into our regular eating routines.

We have looked at the fundamentals of mindful eating in this guide, such as being aware of the present moment, observing without passing judgment, and paying attention to signals of hunger and fullness. We've also talked about how to incorporate mindful eating into other facets of daily life and how to overcome typical obstacles.

Adopting a more intuitive and holistic approach to eating is what mindful eating is all about, not about adhering to rigid guidelines or regimens. It's about developing appreciation for the sustenance that food offers, appreciating each meal, and listening to our bodies' wisdom.

Let's keep in mind that growth is a journey, not a destination, as we continue on our mindful eating adventure. It's about living in the present and making tiny, lasting adjustments, believing that each conscious decision we make improves our general health and wellbeing.

I pray that we will approach our meals with love, curiosity, and compassion, understanding that mindful eating involves not just what we eat but also how we eat and the significant effects it has on our lives. May mindfulness help us to nourish ourselves with more than just food—may it be a greater sense of joy, connection, and presence.

THE END